The Vocal Pitstop

The Vocal Pitstop

Keeping Your Voice on Track

Adam D. Rubin, M.D.

Contributing Author: Cristina Jackson-Menaldi, Ph.D.
Cover art and original illustrations: David Cascardo

Forewords by Melissa Errico & Ron Livingston

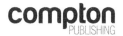

This edition first published 2014 © 2014 by Compton Publishing Ltd.

Registered office: Compton Publishing Ltd, 30 St. Giles', Oxford,

OX1 3LE, UK Registered company number: 07831037

Editorial offices: 3 Wrafton Road, Braunton, Devon, EX33 2BT, UK

Web: www.comptonpublishing.co.uk

ISBN 978-1-909082-13-7

A catalogue record for this book is available from the British Library.

Cover illustration: Daniel Cascardo, http://www.danielcascardo.com

Cover design: David Siddall, http://www.davidsiddall.com

Set in Adobe Caslon Pro 12pt by Stuart Brown

1   2014

Table of Contents

Acknowledgments

Special thanks to my mentors, Drs. Robert Sataloff and Daniel Megler, as well as to all my partners and staff at the Lakeshore Ear, Nose & Throat Center for their continued support. A big thank you to Cristina Jackson-Menaldi, Ph.D. She is truly incredible at her work, and I am thankful for her contributions to this book. Thank you to my friend and talented artist, Daniel Cascardo. If you do not know his work, please visit his website, www.danielcascardo.com. It will blow you away. Thanks to Melissa Errico and Ron Livingston for their touching forwards, my publisher, Noel McPherson, Matthew Chosid, and Alyssa Pajakowski.

Thanks to my entire family, but particularly my parents for supporting me all through my lifetime, particularly when I was the only one of their five children not to go straight into medical school. They never missed a show through my college or professional acting career. My dad was my greatest supporter (and greatest critic). He was a great physician, and I know he would be proud of me for this book and other endeavors. He often reminded me to make sure that I thank him when I received an Oscar or Tony award. That is unlikely to happen at this point, but I am sure this will do.

Lastly, I would like to thank our patients, who give us the privilege of caring for their precious instruments.

To my wife, Rebecca, and two kids, Whitney and Noah, for their constant love and support, and for letting me sing around the house . . .usually.

Foreword

by Melissa Errico

I wish I had read a book like this when I was starting out. Let me back up a little and tell you that I met Dr. Adam Rubin when we were undergraduate students at Yale University and a part of a community of peers that sang and did theater, concerts, cabarets, and acapella harmony groups at every available moment between our other regular studies. To me, he was a singer. We all went on to professional lives in the theater (including Adam!) and eventually I heard he had become a successful throat doctor. How cool, I thought! It is a pleasure to write this foreword for an old friend who loves and knows about music and performance, and who is also now a part of the medical side of the voice.

I've learned a lot about the voice over the years. I started my professional career at age 18 in the First National Tour of *Les Miserables* playing the role of Cosette (in fact, I dropped out of my freshman year at Yale to do this, and returned three semesters later). That was an interesting beginning and perhaps could be something of a cautionary tale in retrospect. When you are on the road, everyone in the cast thinks they are a throat doctor and expert. This is probably true of any group of actors in a show, talking freely backstage about this or that health condition. I remember people 'curing' each other of colds with herbal remedy suggestions (often bad ideas), travel steamers (good), Advil for hoarseness (not good at ALL), Mucinex (fine, but if you don't drink enough water, not great), etc., etc. Some people warmed up. Some people did not. Some people partied and drank each night. Some were very disciplined. I was so young and extremely conscientious. I remember loving the show, being amazed by the gorgeous music, adoring the character of Cosette – and finding the lifestyle of professional performing somewhat lonely. I also realized how confusing it was to wade through all the unofficial 'advice' from my fellow actors. Eight shows a week takes so much focus, and so much maintenance of sleep and food. I managed the singing requirements of Cosette, leaning on several years of good vocal training and probably a good deal of natural intuition (not to mention youth!). I found it very hard to unwind at night after each show. There was so much excitement in the experience, but then so much importance placed on rest and recovery, sometimes made harder by traveling and setting up temporary homes. I never knew when to eat dinner and I ate after the shows. (I hadn't heard of reflux YET.) I gained a ton of weight until we arrived in Detroit and I signed up for a local diet center and learned about eating protein, regular meals, and plenty of vegetables. As well as slimming down to my very best, I noticed a big change in my energy and my sense of confidence. By the time I returned to college, I had much better habits than the average pizza-at-midnight student.

As time went on, I did many Broadway musicals. I cannot go into all the lessons learned, but I do recall my second Broadway show playing Eliza Doolittle in *My Fair Lady* at the age of 22. That was a role that suited my voice perfectly – as I had always had an easy middle voice with a lot of power (good for the urchin) and was a romantic soprano (wishfully) modeled on the sweet feel of Julie Andrews. But, one day, before we opened, I was asked to go to a sound studio to record screaming. The director's concept had a nightmarish element where the audience hears the poor scared Eliza screaming wildly off stage, frightened of what is happening, afraid to become naked to a take a bath, terrified overall of Higgins' experiment. So, without complaint, I went to the studio after a full day of work and screamed for over ten minutes, giving the sound engineer lots of choices. The next morning, I was hoarse and I knew something was wrong. I had a vocal hemorrhage. Eventually, it was surgically repaired. Needless to say, I learned that there are certain extreme requests that we as singers sometimes shouldn't fulfil. Yes, I wish I hadn't screamed. But in the end, I relied on good medical care and pulled through. When it opened, the *New York*

Times said 'Newcomer Melissa Errico is beguiling'. I was grateful to be singing and healthy again and not too worried about being beguiling, though that was nice to hear!

Reading *The Vocal Pitstop*, I was struck by the way we learn things. We *should* actually have a plan, and not go about the process guessing. When we are very young, we don't know exactly who could teach the whole picture – the actual singing of music, finding a connection to songs and characters (an emotional journey in itself), as well as the medical and health aspects. I had voice lessons growing up, but the nature of being a teenager is a lot of flux, travel, going to college, and it is hard to get any consistency. During *My Fair Lady*, I found a voice teacher in New York City who I have stayed with until this very day. I go every Wednesday at 1 PM. And have for 20 years. In my 20s, I married Patrick McEnroe, a professional tennis player. I was struck by how similar his life was to mine. We are both athletes. Singing is like sports and setbacks are a natural part of it all. Injuries do happen, for whatever reason, and we address them and heal. Now, I am a mother to three young daughters, and new challenges exist (and new inspiration for sure!). I juggle motherhood with my love of theater and singing. I have made records, done more musicals, plays and TV, and enjoy touring with symphonies in concert. I am mindful to get enough sleep, not to talk too loud with three boisterous kids, to do yoga and stay fit.

Little details have become a part of my discipline. The importance of warming up, of course, but we also must *cool down* our voices. It's very hard to do, but we cannot chat with the audience after the show, or go out socializing with all the beloved guests and family who come to see performances. In the book you are about to read, you will read about the voice on a very practical level – how it works, how to protect it, and how to approach a professional career. Especially for singers just starting out, I think this book is invaluable. For anyone who needs their voices strong and free, which really is everyone, there is something to learn here.

Enjoy those voices. Your voice. Stay healthy and stay calm.

Thank you Dr. Adam Rubin for using your voice to support all those who will benefit from your writing. I know I'll keep a copy in my own dressing room.

Foreword

by Ron Livingston

Wow! Adam Rubin has written the definitive owner's manual for the professional voice. With pictures.

When I first met Adam at Yale in the late 80s, he was an actor, director, and baritone for the acappella Society of Orpheus and Bacchus. Together, we studied voice work, scene beats, and how to be present, honest, and compelling on stage. He directed me in class as one of history's more unlikely Stanley Kowalskis, and a year later was truly magnificent playing Lopakhin in my thesis production of *The Cherry Orchard*. Adam Rubin was the consummate dedicated performer.

Then we graduated and I heard conflicting reports that he was either working off-Broadway, touring in *Oklahoma!*, or going to Harvard Medical School. Turns out they were all true.

With *Vocal Pitstop*, Adam – sorry, make that Dr. Adam D. Rubin, M.D. – has now drawn upon his unique perspective as an actor, singer, and leading laryngologist to create an *indispensable* guide for anyone who relies on their voice to make a living. It should be required reading in any conservatory or communications program, and I selfishly wish he'd written it twenty-five years ago. Except then I'd have missed out on one hell of a Lopakhin. So let's just say I'm very, very grateful to have it now.

Preface

As a laryngologist who was a former working actor and singer, I am thrilled to have the opportunity to write this book. When I was in high school, college, and acting professionally, like many other performers, I had little knowledge about how to recognize, avoid, evaluate, and manage vocal injuries. I blindly used homeopathic remedies that another performer, singing teacher, or even physician might have suggested without really knowing the nature of my injury or cause of my hoarseness. I still remember loading up on aspirin during a run of a show, because one of my coworkers told me it would reduce inflammation to the vocal folds. He failed to mention it would increase my risk for vocal fold hemorrhage. In high school, I played Horace Vandergelder in *Hello, Dolly!* I was becoming progressively hoarser through using a 'character voice' to sound older. I had essentially no voice by opening night. Believe it or not, a doctor told me to gargle with Jack Daniels and terpin hydrate with codeine. I have no idea how he convinced my father, an excellent physician, to follow those instructions. I feel very fortunate that that was not the end of my singing career right there and then.

I, like others, often lived in denial or assumed my hoarseness would resolve with time. On the other hand, I also lived in fear that my voice would not be in prime shape when called upon to perform. I had never heard of videostroboscopy, let alone knew who out there in the medical profession specialized in professional voice care or what made for an appropriate evaluation of the voice. This is a desperately needed book for the performer to have and even carry with them to auditions, on tours, backstage, or to the doctor's office. But it is not only for the high-end performer; it will help anyone who values or depends on a healthy voice for their livelihood or happiness. This handbook is a fairly concise reference explaining in fairly simple terms how the voice works, what can go wrong, how to avoid serious career-threatening injury, where to seek help, how to stay working when things are not perfect, and when it is necessary to shut things down. In a sense, this book is a chance to share with others my own 'if I only knew then what I know now'. I hope you enjoy it.

Adam D. Rubin, M.D.
www.lakeshoreent.com
@VoiceDocintheD

Introduction
Why do I need this book?

'I thought it was my allergies.' 'I thought my laryngitis would get better in a couple of days.' 'I knew I was hoarse, but I was still able to perform reasonably well.' These are all variations on themes commonly heard from patients who suffer a voice change, but wait longer than they should to be appropriately evaluated. Perhaps they finally come in when they realize their upper range has not returned in months; or they cannot get through the day teaching without losing the voice. The delay may be due to denial, or, more likely, to not realizing that voice change may be the sign of something more serious.

The voice is a precious and delicate instrument. It is one of our most effective, if not our most accessible, means of communicating and expressing ourselves. We use it on a daily basis, and yet often take it for granted, thinking it will always be there when we need it. Many consider some degree of hoarseness as expected or acceptable. Fortunately, most vocal injuries will resolve themselves given our bodies' ability to heal. However, this is not always the case. A delay in identifying the problem and providing appropriate treatment can prevent normal voice recovery and leave someone significantly impaired. Anyone who has lost his or her voice for a significant period of time knows how difficult life can be without it. Maybe it interferes with your social life, your family, or your sense of self. Maybe it interferes with your livelihood. Maybe it is a sign of a major medical problem, even cancer.

Prevention of vocal injury is tantamount to the performer, as he or she might be called upon at any moment and must be in optimal voice. An audition may come through; a last minute gig may be offered; a chance to sing a solo in the high school choir may present itself; a big-time reviewer might be coming to see an evening performance after a brilliant all-out performance in the matinee earlier that day;

a stadium might be sold out awaiting the show. But, the singer or actor is not the only professional dependent on a healthy voice.

What about the teacher working 8-hour days, 5 days a week, then needing to go through parent conferences; the priest or rabbi leading a congregation for the third service of the day; the lawyer making closing arguments to the jury; the doctor talking to patients throughout the day; the soccer coach trying to manage his team; the assembly line leader needing to bellow orders over a noisy environment. Other professions might not demand the same level of vocal quality as the singer, but still demand a serviceable voice that is sustainable. As voice specialists, we see such people almost daily who are concerned they are losing their ability to perform their job.

Although most singers and performers have a keen awareness of their vocal quality and demands, many of them still take the voice for granted. Many acknowledge the importance of training and technique, but still others go on god-given talent, assuming that the voice will always be present in top shape when needed. Even among well-trained performers, few truly understand exactly what makes and keeps the voice working. In addition, when the voice is not all together present, when range is lost or the tone has changed, many will just accept that they have 'laryngitis' without recognizing that a more significant problem may be present.

Some vocal injuries, if not recognized and treated immediately, can have serious career-threatening long-term effects. On the other hand, any performer will likely run into some hoarseness at various points during a run. When should you let an understudy go on? When should you go on voice rest? When should you be seen by a physician? Whom should you see? What can you do to avoid missing work?

Career longevity depends on a healthy voice for many people. The informed voice user should be best prepared to stay healthy, recognize vocal injury, and seek the appropriate attention needed. It would be great to have a quick reference to help prevent and recognize injuries, and help decide what steps should be taken if voice quality changes. A 'pitstop', if you will, for voice maintenance.

The goal of *The Vocal Pitstop* is to provide a source of information that will help the serious (or not quite so serious) voice user enjoy his or her full vocal potential. Years of research have been devoted to explaining the complexity of the human voice. Numerous theories, mathematical equations, and principles of physics contribute to this understanding. This book will speak of none of them. Rather, it will help you keep your voice in the best shape possible; to recognize voice problems; and to know what to do should problems arise. I have even included a flowchart at the back of the book for a quick guide on what to do and where to turn when things go wrong. It will refer you to the appropriate chapter in the book for more details – but do also read the whole book for continuity.

The book is not a substitute for investing in vocal training and working on technique, but will provide you with numerous tips and exercises to help strengthen, preserve, and recover the voice. It is meant for the high-end singer, the young high school performer, the teacher, the coach, and almost anyone else who loves to use his or her voice or depends on it financially. Regardless of what you do, you will likely find usefulness in this book – unless, of course, you are a mime artist.

When a Formula 1 driver feels his car is not operating at full potential he pulls in for a pitstop. When your voice is not functioning at its full potential, you need a vocal pitstop. This book is meant to be that 'pitstop' – to help you:

- understand how your voice works
- recognize when a problem arises
- identify what might be wrong
- be aware of when it is time to bring it in to a 'garage' for service
- know who should provide that service and with what tools

- learn how to keep it going when you are low on gas
- know when you need to stop and turn the engine off.

Do not let your motor fail! Do not blow a gasket! Stop in for routine maintenance and keep your voice running smoothly.

Chapter 1
How do I know if something is wrong with my voice?

The answer to this question is pretty obvious. Any change in the quality of your voice signifies that something has happened to the vocal apparatus. In truth, it is unrealistic to believe that the heavy voice user will never become hoarse. We all know people who seem to have 'cords of steel' (Figure 1a). This may mean they have a genetic makeup of collagen that is more resistant to injury. Of course, it could also mean they have impeccable technique and vocal habits. Ironically, this is not a great name for resilient vocal folds (cords) (Figure 1b) because steel does not vibrate very well.

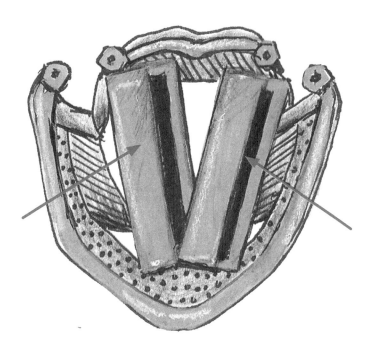

Figure 1a: This picture shows what 'cords of steel' would look like …. good for a paperweight, but will not vibrate very well. Red arrows point to the fictional 'cords of steel'. Compare to Figure 1b.

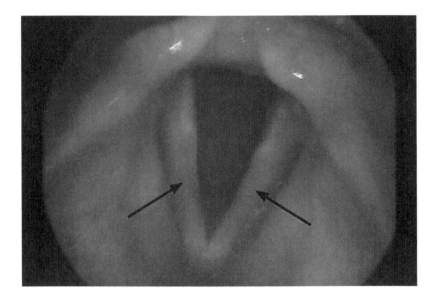

Figure 1b: This picture shows real vocal folds (they actually show my vocal folds). The black arrows point to them. This is the view you would obtain by chopping off the head at the neck and looking down towards the toes – though we would not recommend looking at them that way! We have better, less invasive methods ☺. The vocal folds are housed in the thyroid cartilage in the neck. This cartilage structure is quite prominent in men and is often called the 'Adam's Apple'.

In any case, even the performer with the most resilient of voices will likely run into problems at some point. At the very least, a cold or other upper respiratory infection will predispose someone to hoarseness. However, if you 'know' your voice and can recognize what is different about it, and you have some idea of how the vocal mechanism works, you can get a good idea about what might be happening even without being able to see your vocal folds. Most important to recognize is that not all hoarseness equals 'laryngitis'. Laryngitis implies inflammation to the vocal folds, just as arthritis signifies inflammation to a joint. Although inflammation is a common cause of hoarseness, it is not the only cause. Failure to recognize that can lead to serious long-term vocal problems.

HOARSENESS ≠ LARYNGITIS

We call the vocal 'cords' *vocal folds*. The term 'fold' is more appropriate, because it is a multi-layered structure. The multi-layer architecture gives the vocal fold its ability to vibrate. See Appendix I.

The vocal folds primarily have to do two things: close and vibrate (actually, they also have to open so you can breathe ... that is pretty important too). They are the strings of the vocal instrument. Just like the strings on a violin, they can vibrate at different frequencies to create different pitches. Each violin string has its own thickness, and its frequency can be altered by lengthening or shortening the string. The frequency of vibration of the vocal folds is determined by their thickness, length, and tension. This is controlled by the synchronized activity of a bunch of little muscles within the voice box. The vocal folds are able to vibrate because they are a multi-layered structure with a nice pliable cover. If you want a bit more detail about this, please see Appendix I at the end of this book. Anything that prevents or impairs the vibration of the vocal folds (makes the cover stiffer) will lead to a raspy voice.

A raspy voice is what most people equate to 'hoarseness', but in truth, any change in vocal quality can be considered 'hoarse'.

Sometimes vibratory impairment and resulting voice changes are subtle. The voice just might not 'feel' right. Perhaps it feels like more effort to produce the desired quality of sound. The voice may 'break' or 'crack' frequently. The passagio (or change from chest to head voice) is *very* sensitive to impaired vibration of the vocal folds and voice breaks will often occur within it.

Increased stiffness will also likely be heard more in the upper range of the voice. That is because the vocal fold becomes stretched to produce higher notes. When it is stretched, the nice pliable cover naturally becomes stiffer. So, any additional stiffness will be heard more in the upper pitches. The best way to test this is to sing softly in the upper

One good way to test the health of your vocal folds is to do a glissando (slide from the lowest note to your highest note) on an /ah/ vowel, mezzo piano (fairly quietly). If the voice breaks in that area (and it did not use to), there is likely some increased stiffness to the vocal fold affecting vibration.

range. It is important to sing softly, because anyone can 'blow through' some stiffness and make the vocal folds vibrate by singing loudly.

Of course, the strings on a violin do not vibrate on their own. To make sound one needs to bow across them. The same is true for the vocal folds, but the 'bow' for the voice is the breath. Now one recognizes that breath is not enough to make the vocal folds produce sound. If it was, we would hear voice every time we exhaled. Fortunately, that is not the case or the world would be an even noisier place. Rather, the vocal folds must close to create a seal under which air (breath) pressure can build up and eventually blow the edges of the vocal folds open and start them vibrating (Figure 2).

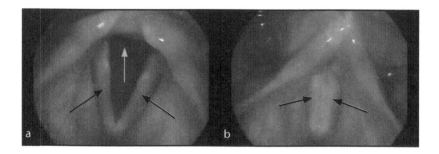

Figure 2a: This picture shows the vocal folds open. They open so that air can get into your lungs when you breathe. **b:** This picture shows the vocal folds closed. They close so that air pressure can build up beneath them and make them vibrate. The black arrows point to the vocal folds. The blue arrow shows the direction of air passing through the vocal folds into the trachea ('wind-pipe'), going to the lungs, when the vocal folds are open.

As the stream of air continues to flow through the closed vocal folds, the vibration is perpetuated. A number of physics principals not worth trying to remember are involved here. One is Bernoulli's principle, which is also involved in airplanes being able to lift off the ground.

Anything that impairs closure of the vocal folds will result in air escape and a breathy quality to the voice. The breathiness may be accompanied by raspiness, because if the vocal folds do not close well that will lead to irregularities in vibration too. When vocal fold closure is severely impaired, you may even feel winded when speaking or singing due to excessive air escape. You may have difficulty projecting as well, as loudness is created by increased air pressure. When the vocal folds do not close it becomes more difficult to build pressure below them.

Back to the violin . . . if you put the same strings on a $100 violin and compared them to what they sound like on a Stradivarius (a *bit* more of an expensive violin!), the sound would be dramatically different. This is because the string is just the source of the sound. What resonates and filters the sound, amplifying different harmonics (overtones), is the body of the violin. This brings out the unique color and tone of each violin. In the human body, the resonator or filter of the sound is the 'vocal tract'. This includes all the space above the vocal folds. The sound is filtered as it passes through the throat, nose, sinuses, and mouth. It is also shaped by the articulators, including the tongue and lips (Figure 3).

So, anything that affects the vocal tract will affect the tone and resonation of the voice. A fairly easy example to understand would be when the nose becomes congested, and the voice becomes hyponasal ('nasally', like when you pinch your nostrils closed).

Lastly, and less commonly, one may hear peculiar sounds to the voice: a tight or intensely strained sound quality, for example. The whole voice apparatus is controlled by the central nervous system (e.g. your brain). Some of this is voluntary (you control it consciously), some is

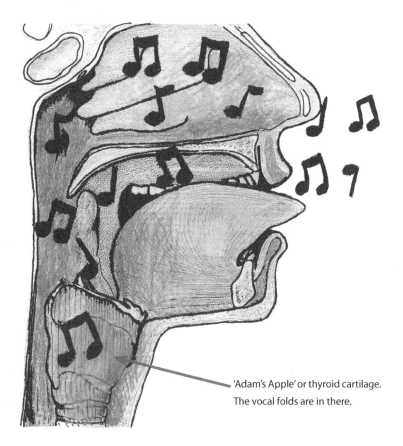

'Adam's Apple' or thyroid cartilage.
The vocal folds are in there.

Figure 3: The illustration above shows the 'vocal tract' or the resonators of the sound. The picture is viewed as if we sliced someone's head right down the middle. We can see the sound coming from the larynx, going upwards and outwards, resonating in the throat, mouth, and nose, and coming out between the lips.

involuntary (reflexes). Sometimes a peculiar quality of the voice can be explained by a neurologic or psychiatric problem. The voice is strongly connected to the psyche and can be affected under periods of great strain or trauma. Other times, the voice may be strained due to poor compensation for another underlying vocal problem, or just due to poor technique.

Ultimately, you should have a keen sense of awareness of your voice – not only the quality, but the body's sensations producing it. Some problems are less obvious than others. Some things to consider: Do things seem more effortful? Is there pain? Is my voice fatiguing more easily? Any such changes may be signs of a vocal problem. Early recognition of a voice problem is important to give yourself the optimal chance of recovering the voice and for identifying any significant medical issue that could be presenting itself through the voice.

Chapter 2
What can go wrong?

Ok, so now you know any change in voice quality merits attention. You also know that a raspy voice means an impairment in vibration; a breathy voice means an impairment in closure; a change in resonance means something awry in the vocal tract; and a peculiar sound to the voice might signify a technical problem or a neurological or psychological issue. Other problems might include a loss of range, decreased vocal stamina, and pain. Well, this chapter will introduce you to what specifically can cause these changes. It is not meant to scare you (well, ok, maybe a little). You need to be aware of what kind of things can go wrong so you are well-informed and can best take care of your instrument. An informed mind is a prepared mind . . . or something like that.

Let's think of the 'categories' of voice changes discussed in the previous chapter.

The **Raspy** Voice

This is by far the most common vocal quality of which performers complain. Now, mind you, some people's voices are naturally raspy and that does not mean there is a problem (otherwise, Bruce Springsteen would not have had such continued success). When a voice becomes raspy or raspier, however, that is the signal that something has changed in the vocal fold architecture. It might not stand in isolation. A voice can be both raspy and breathy, as we will discuss below. But, as you now know, a raspy voice means something is hindering vocal fold vibration. Below are some problems that can do just that.

Inflammation

Inflammation of the vocal folds is 'laryngitis'. Laryngitis will cause raspiness to the voice, but again, one should never assume that raspiness is caused only by inflammation. Infection is a common cause of laryngitis. *Viral laryngitis* occurs during an upper respiratory infection (for example, a cold). The voice will disappear for no other apparent reason besides the cold. *Bacterial laryngitis* can occur as well, but is much less common. Viral laryngitis does not require antibiotics, while bacterial laryngitis does. Viral laryngitis should be distinguished from voice loss that occurs during an upper respiratory infection due to severe coughing. Cough is produced essentially by slamming the vocal folds together, then blowing them open with tremendous force. This can be quite traumatic to the vocal folds, causing a *traumatic laryngitis*. Abusing or misusing the vocal folds can also cause a traumatic laryngitis. The inflammation can persist, particularly if the abusive behavior or overuse continues or the voice is not given time to recover. This is often a problem when a performer has eight shows to do in a week and does not have time to let the inflammation settle down. Inflamed vocal folds are vulnerable to longer lasting injuries. Other things that can cause inflammation of the voice box include: acid reflux, allergies, inhalants (e.g. smoke), medications, and some underlying medical conditions.

Lesions

Any mass or growth on the edge of the vocal fold will impair vibration and result in raspiness. In the context of the performer, most masses are a result of vocal trauma or overuse. These would include nodules, polyps, cysts, pseudocysts, and fibrotic masses (Figure 4). Discussion of each of these masses is more than you need to know at this point, but suffice it to say that some of these masses will go away with voice therapy, while others may require surgery. Other masses can form without vocal trauma including papillomas (warty growths) and cancer.

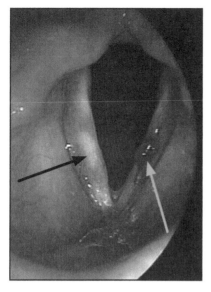

Figure 4: The black arrow points to a white cyst underneath the surface of the vocal fold. The blue arrow points to blood within the vocal fold (hemorrhage) which is shaping into a polyp. The young woman was told for years that her voice was hoarse due to her allergies. No one had identified the large cyst within her vocal fold. The polyp is likely a more recent development given the presence of fresh blood. If identified earlier, the cyst would have been smaller and easier to remove. The polyp likely would have been avoided altogether. Now, both vocal folds require surgical intervention

Hemorrhage

A vocal fold hemorrhage (Figure 4) is a bleed into the substance of the vocal fold. It occurs when a blood vessel within the vocal fold ruptures. This is usually the result of a vocally traumatic event: straining, screaming, or coughing, for example. If hemorrhages are not recognized and treated appropriately, they can turn into polyps, or worse, scar.

Vocal fold hemorrhage and tear are two indications for absolute voice rest – which means being pulled off stage and missing work if necessary.

Vocal fold tear

This, too, is a result of a traumatic insult to the vocal folds. It is analogous to biting the inside of the lip. It results in significant surrounding inflammation and stiffness. If improperly treated it can lead to development of a mass or scar (Figure 5).

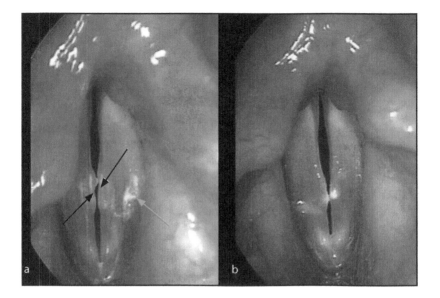

Figure 5a: The vocal folds of a singer who was hoarse two days after a three-set gig. The black arrows point to swellings or masses at the edge of each vocal fold, with what look like small 'cookie-bites'. These are mucosal tears. Notice how red and inflamed the vocal folds are, with some patches of mucus present (blue arrow), another sign of inflammation. **b** The same singer after two days of voice rest and steroid treatment. The vocal folds are less inflamed and red, the swellings have gone down in size, and the 'cookie-bite' appearance is less prominent. The mucosal tears are healing. Hopefully, the singer will be left with smooth edges once completely healed. This singer is also given voice therapy to help rehabilitate the vocal folds.

Scar

Scar is a four-letter word in the area of voice. Scar involves losing some or all of Reinke's space – the most pliable layer of the vocal folds (see Appendix I). This can result in severe stiffness of the vocal fold. To date, we still have no great treatment for scar, so efforts should be made to avoid developing it. The severity of the problem will depend on the severity of the scar. Furthermore, scarring of both vocal folds will result in a much worse voice than scarring of only one vocal fold (Figure 6).

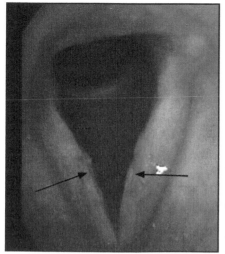

Figure 6: Vocal folds of a teacher and athletic coach who had become progressively hoarse for many years. It was getting to the point where she could not use her voice for more than 15 minutes, before she nearly lost it completely. The arrows point to deep craters on the edge of each vocal fold. These 'craters' are where the tissue layer below the epithelium (Reinke's space) has been obliterated. The epithelium (epithelium is basically the 'skin' of the vocal fold) is tacked down to the deeper layers of the vocal fold. This is a severe scar that will not vibrate well. This is a tough problem that could have been avoided if she had come for help when she initially started having voice problems.

Poor breath support

'Breath support' is a term thrown around a lot. Ultimately, one needs to provide a steady stream of airflow through the vocal folds without running out of air too quickly or intermittently cutting off the flow so as to disrupt the sound. The volume (power) of the voice is going to be affected, and should be controlled by the amount of pressure supplied by the breath. This should be controlled by flow, not by 'muscling' the sound. Precisely coordinating breath with voicing is key to healthy phonation. Compromised breath support from asthma, emphysema, rib cage injuries or abnormalities, and poor technique can affect vocal fold vibration.

The **Breathy** Voice

The vocal folds are able to open and close because they are attached to cartilage which rotates on a joint. The joint is moved by the small muscles within the voice box which are activated by nerves (Appendix I). Poor closure of the vocal folds may be due to injury to the nerves or joints which move the vocal folds or from something structural getting in the way. When the vocal folds do not close appropriately, this results in a breathy voice.

Vocal fold paralysis or paresis

Injury to the nerves which move the vocal folds will lead to poor closure and a breathy voice. One of the most common causes of injury to the nerves to the vocal fold is surgery in the neck, such as thyroid or cervical spine surgery. Anyone having these types of surgeries should be aware that such a complication (which can occur even in the hands of the best surgeon), can be voice and career threatening. One should make sure that the surgery is necessary and the potential benefits outweigh this risk. Vocal fold paralysis can also be caused by a virus and other disease processes . . . even cancer.

Lesions

A large enough mass on the edge of the vocal fold will impair closure as well as vibration. As a result, the voice will sound raspy *and* breathy.

Scar

If scarring is severe enough it can affect the closure of the vocal folds. Again, the voice will sound raspy *and* breathy.

Poor breath support

Poor breath support can also affect closure.

Loss of range

Impaired vibration

Anything that impairs vibration will result in loss of range. This is because in order to reach higher pitches, the vocal fold stretches and becomes tighter. So, the cover of the fold naturally becomes stiffer and anything that causes additional stiffness may prevent the vocal fold from vibrating at the higher frequencies. The passagio (the transition between vocal registers) is a *very* sensitive area affected by vocal fold stiffness. When there is impaired vibration, one will likely have a significant 'break' in the passagio. Again, this can be tested by sliding from a low to high note fairly softly.

Injury to the superior laryngeal nerve

This nerve is a small nerve, but is responsible for stretching the vocal fold to obtain higher pitches. Permanent injury to this nerve can be disastrous for a singer's career. It is particularly at risk during thyroid surgery.

Poor breath support

Poor breath support will result in decreased ability to vibrate vocal folds that are more tensioned, resulting in inability to hit higher notes.

Change in resonance

Change in resonance results from a change in the resonators above the vocal folds. The most common cause would be nasal congestion from allergies or a cold. Other things that could affect resonance include polyps in the nose, tonsillitis, other growths in the throat, poor soft palate movement after a stroke or other neurological event, and surgery on any part of the vocal tract.

Peculiar sounds

Peculiar sounds, such as severely strained voice quality, are often the result of a neurological or psychological problem. These are beyond the scope of this book.

Throat pain

Throat pain should be evaluated by a physician. However, pain that comes about only during voice use is likely a sign of an underlying voice problem. It may be secondary to excessive muscle tension during voice production. This excessive tension may be due to compensation for another voice problem or from poor technique. Sometimes, one can develop muscular inflammation and tendinitis involving the muscles surrounding the larynx. Throat pain during voicing may also be a sign of an injury to the vocal fold(s).

Chapter 3
Should I stop working?

This is a very difficult dilemma for a performer in the middle of a run encountering a change in vocal quality (Figure 7). Of course, it is also a dilemma for the teacher debating whether to call in the substitute. A number of considerations come into play:

1. Am I causing myself permanent injury?
2. Will my income suffer?
3. Will they think I am too fragile if I take time off?
4. Will I hurt my future by not sounding my best if I continue to perform?
5. Will it hurt my fan base if I cancel a show?

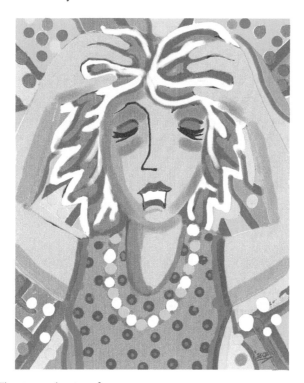

Figure 7: The stressed out performer.

There is always a need to balance short-term concerns with long-term concerns. First and foremost, however, you must determine if you have caused a vocal fold hemorrhage or tear, because these are two absolute indications for voice rest. Using the voice in either of those cases puts you at risk for mass, or worse, scar formation. This can be career threatening. Let me say that again: *career threatening*. Unfortunately, finding out if you have one of these problems requires an appropriate evaluation (discussed in Chapter 5). A significant hemorrhage might mean being pulled off stage or out of work for as much as six weeks, while a tear might mean being pulled off stage for just a few days. If there is no hemorrhage or tear, but rather inflammation from overuse or an upper respiratory infection, efforts should be made to do whatever must be done medically to preserve and recover the voice, and to prevent further injury.

Some questions to ask yourself are:

1.   *Can I perform despite my hoarseness?*
This will depend on several factors. For example, are you a coloratura performing 'Queen of the Night', or do you just have a cameo speaking role? What are your vocal responsibilities? What type of music do you sing? How pristine does the quality of the voice have to be?

2.   *Can I do anything to make the performance less taxing?*
For example, can I change melodies? Can I use or rely more on amplification?

3.   *Can I perform well?*
There is always a balance between looking undependable versus the risk of having a bad performance. This is a delicate decision and requires some real soul-searching.

4. Can I perform without hurting myself more?

It does no good to belt your way through a performance only to find yourself more compromised the next day. You may end up missing more performances than you would have if you had let your under-study go on for a day or two. Do *not* let your ego get in the way of making a wise decision! Signs that things are getting worse include: worsening sound quality, loss of range, increased throat pain, and increased vocal fatigue.

5. What will happen if I do not perform?

Can someone else step in and take your place? Will the show/gig have to be cancelled? You have to think about your personal health, but should also consider the ramifications of not performing.

6. Is there anything I can do to keep me on stage?

To answer this, see the next chapter!

One must always weigh short-term goals against long-term goals and career longevity. This is not always easy. An actor who pulls himself off-stage for a few performances in a row, could find him- or her-self replaced permanently. On the other hand, causing a more serious injury could threaten the rest of an actor's career.

Chapter 4
I can't stop working, what should I do?!

Rest

Resting the voice is important for voice recovery. This does not necessarily mean absolute voice rest, but in general a good principle is to rest the voice when you don't need to be using it. You might think of it as 'rest the voice if you are not getting paid for it'. In other words, avoid getting on the cell phone in the car. Avoid excessive talking after a performance. Avoid loud environments after a performance. Don't talk off-stage. *A list of do's and don'ts is found Appendix II*. Ultimately, you must take your vocal hygiene to a whole new level, although many of these principles should be followed routinely!

Performance modification

Whatever you can do to make the performance less taxing and challenging can help. This is often easier for the rock singer performing several sets in a bar or someone singing his or her own music. A singer in an opera or musical is going to have less freedom in altering the script, libretto, or melodies. Here are a few suggestions:

1. Reconsider your repertoire. Sing the songs well within your range and avoid more vocally challenging pieces.
2. Check any excess effort at the door. Many actors give 200% during a performance. See how little effort is required to give a great performance. In fact, you may realize you can give an even more effective performance if you 'push' less and 'sink' into the role.
3. Change melodies to make the song less taxing.

4. Use amplification if you have not been. If you have been using it, lean on your amplification a bit more. Take advantage of it. A little reverberation effect can be helpful too. ☺

5. Save your voice during group numbers. Learn to mouth the words well without any vocal effort. Do not waste your vocal reserve on group numbers when you are not absolutely needed. This is important for singers in a choir. Same goes with back-up singing. If you are the lead singer of the band, but sing back-up on a few numbers, conserve on those tunes.

Medications

Some medications can be useful in the appropriate situation to help recover the voice. One should consult a physician before starting any medications, including over-the-counter medications.

Prednisone (a steroid) is a powerful anti-inflammatory and is excellent medication for rapidly reducing vocal fold inflammation. Unfortunately, like many medications it has the potential for bad side-effects. One always needs to weigh potential benefits and risks in every medical decision. In any case, while prednisone can be very helpful, it should only be used on rare occasions and for a short period of time. There are other steroids besides prednisone. Steroids can be given by injection (for the most rapid effect) or as a pill. If you are requiring steroids for your voice too frequently, it means you are doing something fundamentally wrong. This needs to be addressed with training, voice therapy, or other means. Steroids should only be prescribed by a physician.

Lozenges can be soothing for the voice and throat. Glycerin-based lozenges are likely best. Avoid lozenges with menthol and any others which have a numbing effect on the throat. Sensation is important for feedback when using the voice. Anesthetizing the throat may increase your risk for further injury.

Anti-reflux medications are useful medications to help vocal folds heal even if you do not get heartburn. Even a drop or two of acid can cause injury to the vocal folds, particularly when they are already compromised. Creating a healthy environment for vocal folds to heal is important.

Topical nasal decongestants such as oxymetazoline may be useful for significant nasal congestion in the setting of a cold. However, they should be used only for a few days as they can have a rebound effect resulting in physical addiction.

Nasal steroid sprays can be helpful for people with chronic nasal congestion due to allergies.

Nasal saline rinses and sprays like Sinus Rinse and Neti Pot are great for cleaning out the nasal passages. You should use only distilled water when mixing the salt water packets. Do not use tap water.

Cough suppressants and **mucus thinners** such as guaifenesine and dextromorphan are over-the-counter medications that help thin secretions and suppress cough. These can be quite useful, particularly when one has a cold. If these are not sufficient, stronger cough suppressants can be prescribed by a physician.

Dr. Gould's Gargle is a natural home-made concoction that can be soothing and help thin secretions.

Dr. Gould's Gargle

½ teaspoon kosher or pickling salt

½ teaspoon baking soda

½ teaspoon honey or corn syrup

8 oz warm water.

Gargle for 15–20 seconds, then spit until the concoction is finished.

Beware of homeopathic over-the-counter remedies. A number of homeo-pathic remedies are available. Many of them are commercial and can cost quite a bit of money. Most of these have not been studied. They may contain substances which thin the blood and increase risk for vocal fold hemorrhage. They may also be harmful to other parts of your body, such as your kidneys.

Hydration

Hydration, hydration, and more hydration. The vocal folds need to stay well lubricated. Drink lots of water. Sit in the steam of your shower or get a laryngeal steamer.

Vocal exercises

Semi-occluded vocal tract exercises can be useful for voice recovery and are described in Chapter 7. In the setting of the hoarse voice they should be done primarily without sound.

Treatment for throat pain

Throat pain should be evaluated by a physician. However, pain that comes about only during voice use is likely secondary to excessive mus-cle tension during voice production. Sometimes, one can develop mus-cular inflammation and tendinitis involving the muscles surrounding the larynx. Laryngeal massage and voice therapy are often helpful for this. Sometimes, a steroid injection into the affected area can be use-ful. Throat pain can affect the voice, as it will likely affect vocal tech-nique as a performer may 'guard' to prevent worsening of the pain. You should avoid the use of lozenges or sprays that anesthetize the throat, however, if you must perform. Feedback from sensations in the throat is very important to avoid causing further injury during phonation.

Vocal hygiene

Of course, maximizing vocal hygiene becomes all the more important with a compromised voice. See Chapter 6.

Rules for a cold

1. Get plenty of sleep.
2. Speak as little as possible when you do not need to be speaking. Preserve your voice.
3. Hydrate. Drink plenty of water.
4. Cool mist humidifier.
5. Treat your nose (see above).
6. Try to suppress a cough (see above). Keep the cough 'breathy' if unavoidable.
7. Glycerin throat lozenges (avoid menthol or other irritating or numbing lozenges).
8. Tylenol (acetaminophen) to keep your fever down.
9. Recognize your voice limitations.
10. If your voice is hoarse, but you need/want to perform, see a specialist to rule out hemorrhage or tear. Steroids may be useful if there is a viral laryngitis.
11. Be smart. Do not cause yourself a long-term vocal injury by overdoing it.
12. Modify your performance (see previous discussion).

Chapter 5
Where do I find help?

The performer should be aware of how the voice is properly evaluated. For example, a physician putting a tongue depressor in the mouth, looking at the back of the throat while you say 'ah', is not sufficient!

The vocal folds have to be visualized to evaluate hoarseness. The best, and most appropriate, way to evaluate the voice is with a method called 'videostroboscopy', which is described in detail below. It involves using a rigid telescope inserted into the mouth or a flexible scope passed through the nose which allows the clinician to not only see the vocal folds, but to also see them vibrating. A vocal fold can look perfectly straight, but be stiff and not vibrate well. That would be missed without videostroboscopy.

There are a number of people in the medical profession who are most involved with the evaluation of the voice. These include the *laryngologist* and *voice pathologist*.

Laryngology is a subspecialty of *otolaryngology* (or Ear, Nose, and Throat). Although most otolaryngologists have some training in voice care, laryngologists have extra training and expertise in the management of voice disorders.

Voice pathology is a subspeciality of *speech pathology*. Speech pathology includes treatment of all communication disorders as well as swallowing disorders. In other words, speech pathologists may treat problems with articulation, cognitive aspects of communication, language, as well as voice. Voice pathologists have extra training and expertise in evaluating voice disorders and treating them with *voice therapy*. Voice therapy is essentially physical therapy for the injured voice. Therapy is directed at the particular injury or voice problem suffered by the patient. So, having an accurate diagnosis before starting is critical. Ideally, laryngologists and voice pathologists work together as a *voice team* (Figure 8) to evaluate and treat the voice patient. This team may also include the patient's singing teacher, choir director, and other physicians, nurses, and staff involved in the patient's general health. This is typically performed at a voice center. There are a growing number of voice centers throughout the USA, Europe, and the developed world.

It is important to find someone(s) who can appropriately and accurately diagnose your voice problem. Unfortunately, voice subspecialists are not always available. A performer on the road may have to find the best available option. The most important question to answer in the

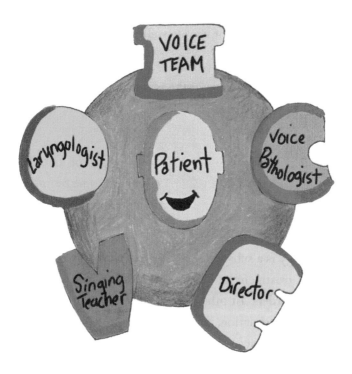

Figure 8: Schematic of a voice team.

acute setting is: Can I continue to perform? Performing on a hemor-rhage or tear can cause permanent, career-threatening damage to the vocal folds.

You should use the internet to search for voice centers near you. If one is not available, a general otolaryngologist should be seen. When the need for care is not emergent (e.g. no pressing engagement), you should feel encouraged to travel to get additional opinions. In addi-tion, you should ask the physician how much voice experience he or she has; how much of his or her practice is geared to the professional voice. This is particularly important if surgery is being recommended. The more subspecialized in voice the physician is, the more experience and skill s/he and her/his voice team will likely have in treating the problem.

What is videostroboscopy?

Videostroboscopy (VS) is a technique to evaluate the structure and vibratory characteristics of the vocal folds. As mentioned and seen below, VS may be performed using a rigid telescope that is moved through the mouth and looks downwards towards the voice box, or a flexible scope which is passed through the nose and also looks down-wards to the vocal folds (Figure 9). This last feat can be accomplished similar to the way the spaghetti noodle trick is performed. Some kids like to pass a spaghetti noodle through their nose and pull it out through their mouth. They are able to do this because the different areas of the vocal tract are all connected.

In any case, a surface microphone is placed on the skin over the larynx. This picks up the frequency of vibration of the vocal folds and sends this information to a computer. The computer in turn tells a strobe light to flash at a speed just slightly slower than the speed of vibra-tion of the vocal folds. As a result, the light flashes at slightly differ-ent points in the vibratory cycle of the vocal fold, yielding a bunch of

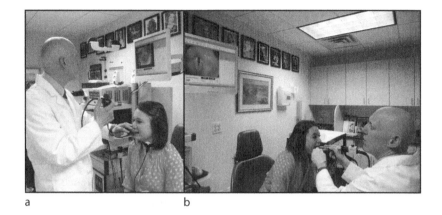

a   b

Figure 9a: In this picture the vocal folds are visualized with a flexible scope through the nose. The surface microphone on the patient's neck will recognize the frequency of vibration of the vocal folds and inform the computer on how fast to flash the strobe light so that vibration can be assessed. **b**: A rigid telescope is inserted into the patient's mouth and the vocal folds are visualized on the screen. Notice how

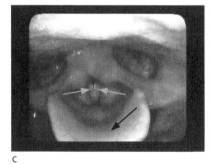

magnified the vocal folds are compared to the picture in which the flexible scope is used. **9c**: Picture of the larynx when visualized with a flexible scope. Notice the difference compared to the pictures in Chapter 1, which were taken with a rigid telescope through the mouth. The black arrow shows the epiglottis. The blue arrows point to the vocal folds.

c

different images to the clinician's eyes. Because the human eye can only perceive still images at speeds well below the frequency of vibration of the vocal folds, the images blend and give the appearance of continuous slow motion. This allows us to assess the vibratory capabilities of the vocal folds and look for areas of stiffness and other abnormalities. This is analogous to the flip book you might have made in your childhood, in which a stick figure is drawn on each page in a slightly different position. When the pages are flipped rapidly, it appears as though the figure is moving.

How fast do the vocal folds vibrate?

Speed of vibration is called 'frequency'. Frequency is a physical parameter of vibration: the rate at which a waveform is repeated per unit of time. It is measured in hertz (Hz), which is defined as cycles/second. The speed of vibration is perceived by the human ear as 'pitch'. Pitch is a perceptual characteristic of sound. The higher the frequency, the higher the pitch. The achievable frequencies of vibration will vary from individual to individual and voice type. Here are some possible ranges for various voice types (musical notes are put in parentheses for those of you interested):

Bass	65–349 Hz (C2–F4)
Baritone	83–440 Hz (E2–A4)
Tenor	98–523 Hz (G2–C5)
Alto	131–784 Hz (C3–G5)
Mezzo Soprano	165–880 Hz (E3–A5)
Soprano	196–1318 Hz (G3–E6)

The flexible laryngoscope (passed through the nose) is an excellent tool for assessing the biomechanics of the larynx as a whole: looking at the opening and closing of the vocal folds, looking for nerve injury and excessive muscle activity. The rigid telescope (passed through the mouth) gives more magnification and allows for identifying more subtle masses and other structural abnormalities. Newer technology for flexible scopes ('distal-chip' technology) has improved the sensitivity of these tools, but still does not provide the magnification of the rigid endoscope.

Knowing what tools are available to evaluate the voice will help you understand whether you are receiving an adequate, sophisticated evaluation of the voice so appropriate diagnosis and recommendations can be made. Knowing you are being evaluated by people who know how to use and interpret these tools is equally important.

A bit about surgery

Surgery on the vocal folds, also called 'microlaryngeal surgery', may be warranted in cases in which voice therapy and medical management are not sufficient to fix the problem. Many are fearful about such surgery because of the well-publicized, unfortunate case of Julie Andrews, one of the greatest singers ever. As with any type of surgery, risks and benefits must be considered. One of the risks of microlaryngeal surgery is worsening of the voice. However, in the right hands this complication is rare. On the other hand, there also may be a risk in *not* doing surgery. For example, if you have a polyp on one vocal fold it can cause significant trauma to the other side. This can lead to another mass on the other vocal fold, or worse, significant scarring which can decrease the ability of the surgeon to recover the voice. We have no great solutions for vocal fold scar. Every surgery has risks, whether it is fixing an injured knee, or removing a mass from a vocal fold. That said, you should feel comfortable asking the surgeon how much experience he or she has with performing microlaryngeal surgery. Also, every case is different. You should be clear about the risks and how much improvement the surgeon expects from the procedure in order to make an informed decision.

Chapter 6
Vocal hygiene: maintaining a healthy voice

The keys to maintaining a healthy voice are:

1. Prevention of vocal injury
2. Recognition of vocal injury
3. Appropriate and timely management of vocal injury to avoid long-term sequelae, particularly vocal fold *scar*.

We have talked about numbers 2 and 3 already in this book. Number 1 depends on understanding the vocal mechanism, getting good training, and good vocal hygiene. The secret of maintaining vocal health is basically: ***Optimizing the use of the resonators and breath support, while minimizing stress on the vocal folds***. In addition to good technique, this requires keeping the vocal folds *and* the whole body healthy.

In this chapter, we discuss basic tips for good 'vocal hygiene'. Adhering to all of these recommendations might lead you to conclude that your life will be boring and limited. It is up to each individual to determine how restrictive he or she must be to maintain his or her vocal health. The high-end performer who needs absolute clarity to his or her voice at any point in the day will likely want to heed the advice more strictly. Nobody said it would be easy . . .

Hydration

The vocal folds like lubrication. Dryness is an enemy of good vibration. Think of water as your engine's lubricant. The voice user should always carry a water bottle, taking frequent sips. A good gauge of hydration is urine color. One should try to maintain 'pale pee'. Darker urine often signifies dehydration. It is possible to drink too much water, but that is unusual. Two to three liters a day is probably a good starting point.

If you exercise or perspire a lot, more is likely required. Drinking a large cup of water as soon as you get up in the morning is a good idea, because you lose fluids during the night.

Hydration with coffee, tea, or soda is less useful, and likely harmful, as they tend to be very acidic and can directly irritate the vocal folds. Also, caffeine is a diuretic. This means it increases water excretion from the body (makes you pee more). If you need that cup of coffee in the morning to 'get you going', drink water after it to rinse the throat. Try to keep your caffeinated beverages to a minimum.

In addition to drinking adequate amounts of water, you should make sure the air around you is adequately humidified. Investment in a humidifier, particularly one that can be used with a furnace, is wise. There are a number of devices sold that deliver steam via inhalation and are good for humidification of the vocal folds. Sitting in a steamy shower can also be useful. With any humidifying device, make sure that filters are changed regularly, and that the air is not 'over-humid-ified' so as to stimulate mold production. A proper level of indoor humidity is 30 to 50%.

Keep your nose moist too! The nose is an important resonator. When it gets dry, it can accumulate crusts which can interfere with resona-tion, as well as get infected and cause post-nasal drainage. Over the counter saline sprays can be useful to keep the nose moist. If you have problems with crusting, the use of a nasal rinse (e.g. Sinus Rinse or Neti Pot) is very useful. Only use distilled water when performing this cleansing (no tap water).

Diet

Yes, what you eat can affect your voice. In general, you want to avoid any diet that increases acid reflux or is directly irritating to the throat. Acid reflux continues to be a hot topic in vocal health. It involves the backwards flow of acid from the stomach into the esophagus and throat. Most people recognize heartburn as reflux, but in fact heartburn is only one symptom of it. When discussing heartburn, one talks about gastroesophageal reflux or GERD. However, other symptoms can be caused by reflux as well. These include the feeling of a lump or mucus in the throat, persistent throat clearing, or even intermittent hoarseness. Although those symptoms are not specific for reflux, when they are present due to acid they are referred to as 'laryngopharyngeal reflux' or 'LPR'. In general, it is risky to assume hoarseness or voice change is from reflux, unless all other potential causes have been ruled out. Many times, someone's hoarseness will be attributed to reflux because the actual cause is missed, such as a small mass, a subtle area of scar, or a nerve weakness.

In any case, reflux can contribute to voice problems. In general, you want to create the healthiest environment for the vocal folds. Controlling acid can be a big part of that. This can be done with dietary and behavioral modifications, and with medications.

Behavioral modifications

1. Elevate the head of your bed with bricks or books under the posts. Do not just use extra pillows or a wedge, as that can increase pressure on your belly and cause reflux.
2. Keep your weight down.
3. Avoid spicy, acidic, tomato-based, or fatty foods like chocolate and fried foods.
4. Limit your intake of caffeinated and acidic drinks, such as coffee, tea, colas, citrus and fruit drinks.
5. Limit your alcohol intake.

Treat your allergies

Allergies can play a role in hoarseness. Nasal congestion can decrease resonation. Allergies may cause swelling at the vocal fold level as well and impair vibration. However, as with reflux, you should never assume hoarseness is from allergies, particularly if there are no other allergy symptoms (e.g. itchy eyes, nasal congestion). Allergy testing is recommended to find out how bad your allergies are and determine what you are allergic to, so you can avoid those things. Allergy medication may be useful, but caution is advised because these medications can cause dryness. A performer with significant allergies should consider immunotherapy (allergy shots).

Suppress the cough

A cough is produced by forceful closure of the vocal folds. Coughing can cause significant injury to the vocal folds. A cough lasting a week should be evaluated by a physician and appropriately treated. If you develop a cough as part of an upper respiratory infection, there are a number of ways to help suppress the cough to avoid vocal trauma (see below). This is particularly important if one has heavy voice obligations.

Medicines

A number of medications can help thin mucus and suppress cough. Some of these are over-the-counter, such as guaifenesin and dextromethorphan, respectively.

Others require a prescription, including codeine and other narcotics, and benzonatate. Obviously, if you have to perform, narcotics are likely not a good idea. Furthermore, benzonatate numbs the throat, and should not be used if you have to perform.

Biofeedback

There are a number of biofeedback techniques that can help suppress cough, called *respiratory retraining*. These can be taught by a speech or voice therapist trained in these techniques. An example of a simple one includes alternating the sound /shhh/ (as though you are telling someone to be quiet in the library), and a 'sniff'. You should sniff with inspiration, then say /shhh/ with expiration. This should be done rapidly, at first. As the urge to cough resolves, the /shhh/ should be elongated and the pattern slowed.

Do not clear your throat

Another type of coughing is throat clearing. This occurs when people feel they have mucus in the throat. They feel it is thick and difficult to bring up. Some people feel the need to clear the throat incessantly. Sometimes, they drive their significant other crazy doing so. Many attribute the sensation to post-nasal drainage. In truth, we see many patients with this complaint, and rarely is it due to true post-nasal drainage. In general, if there is significant mucus on the vocal folds it will be coughed up without too much effort. Generally, this sensation of mucus is caused by irritation of nerve endings within the larynx.

When you clear your throat you bring the vocal folds together with high impact and a potential for damage. Ironically, this can make the sensation of mucus even worse, because it causes more irritation. Instead of clearing, you should try the following:

- Take a sip of water and swallow with your chin down.
- Try to tolerate the sensation in the throat. In other words ignore it, or do not let it get to you. It is unlikely to kill you.
- Produce a 'silent' cough. Just cough with breath coming through, no sound.

The most common cause of this is likely acid reflux. However, it can also be caused by irritation from vocal trauma, neuralgia (irritated nerves from a virus, injury, etc.), allergy, and other even less common etiologies.

Know how your medications affect your voice

A number of medications can affect the voice. Some of these are listed below. If your doctor prescribes these medications, please let him or her know your concerns about your voice. You must weigh the need to take the medications with the potential for harmful effects on the voice.

Anti-histamines: can dry out the vocal folds.

Anti-depressants/psychotropic medications: can dry out the vocal folds.

Diuretics: can dry out the vocal folds.

ACE inhibitors: can cause cough.

Motrin/aspirin/blood thinners: can increase risk for vocal fold hemorrhage.

Calcium channel blockers: can increase gastric reflux.

Hormones/oral contraception: hormones can alter the pitch and quality of the voice. These effects can be permanent. Androgens can lower female voices, for example.

Steroid inhalers: can cause vocal fold inflammation and cause a yeast infection of the vocal folds. If they can be avoided, do so. If you need them to control asthma, make sure you rinse and gargle well with water after each use.

Exercise and maintaining your overall health

Your whole body is involved in voice production. Exercise, eat well, do not smoke or do drugs, and do everything you can to keep yourself in great shape. During exercise, make sure you do not hold your breath. This is a common mistake, particularly when lifting heavy weights. Breath holding is achieved by forcing the vocal folds together, again potentially causing injury. Certainly avoid grunting or other forceful sounds during exercise and other activities (even sex).

A list of 25 tips for a healthy voice is found in Appendix II. Also, see 'Rules for a cold' in Chapter 4.

And, oh yeah . . . **DO NOT SMOKE!** In addition to causing cancer, smoking is extremely irritating to the vocal folds. It causes significant inflammation and can lead to chronic structural changes which can thicken the vocal folds and lower the pitch of the voice (think of Marge Simpson's sisters). It is also damaging to the lining of your nose and respiratory tract, which can result in dryness and crusting; and damages the lungs, resulting in compromised breath support.

Chapter 7
Warming up, cooling down, and everything in-between

Warming up the vocal apparatus before, and cooling it down after, a performance are good ways to improve performance and prevent injury. 'Performance' might mean a day at the office requiring a lot of talking or an opening night on stage. The purpose of this chapter is to provide some basic techniques for warming up and cooling down the voice. For some of you, this may be your first exposure to these types of exercises. Do not let them intimidate you. For those of you with significant vocal training, they are not meant to replace what you have learned and what works for you. You still may find some aspects useful to add to your repertoire. This chapter also cannot substitute for good, supervised vocal training. Everyone's voice, body, and needs are different. Although some of you may find this information sufficient for your vocal needs, it is impossible to personalize technique through a book. If you feel this is sufficient, great, but we would encourage you to search out some degree of hands-on training.

Posture

Your mother always told you to stand up straight. This was likely for cosmetic reasons. She may not have realized she was helping you with healthy voicing as well. Good posture contributes to the strength and health of the voice. It allows for maximal breath support, and reduces tension in muscles we do not want to use as much for voice production. Numerous different techniques have been described, such as the Alexander and Feldenkrais techniques. The individual performer should investigate these techniques and see if they work for him or her. Below are some simple tasks you can try to help improve your posture. Without supervision, please be careful. Listen to your body. Do not try anything that feels uncomfortable.

- Stand with your legs together, the weight of your body centered on your feet.
- Inhale and stretch your arms above your head. Extend your body through your spine to your fingertips.
- Exhale and bend forward, holding the backs of your legs with your hands. Keep your body weight centered and your legs straight.
- Move your forehead towards your legs.
- Hold your breath for 3 seconds, then inhale and straighten up slowly.
- Your ears, shoulders, wrists, hamstrings, and heels should be in alignment. You can use a wall to help (Figure 10).

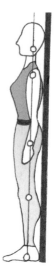

Fig. 10

Relaxation

Relaxation is key to relieving excessive muscle tension that may result in strain on the voice. It also feels great! Life is stressful. We should all look for times to relax. However, a good time to relax is when you are preparing to use your voice. Again, look for techniques that work for you. Massage is a wonderful tool to help the body relax. Some voice therapists and massage therapists are skilled at myofascial release (a technique used to treat muscle pain and tension) of the muscles surrounding the larynx. Such techniques can be useful to maintain or recover a healthy voice. You can even learn to do them yourself. Below is a brief list of things to do to help relax before or after a performance, or any time of day.

- Lie down on the floor with loose clothes and no shoes (Fig.11). Try to relax your body from the top of your head to your toes.
- Gently shake your wrists. Then shake them more vigorously, as if you are trying to get water off of them.
- Move your elbows and hands in a circular manner. 'Wake up' the arms.

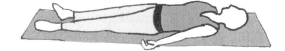

Fig. 11

- Shoulder rolls: Sit or stand straight. Place both of your hands gently on your shoulders with your elbows pointing downward. Inhale and slowly roll your shoulders in a circular manner up and back. Exhale and bring your shoulders forward. Repeat the movement in the opposite direction (Figure 12).
- Neck rolls. Keep your back straight. Drop your chin to your chest and slowly rotate your head in a clockwise direction two or three times. Bring your head back to the center and then gently rotate it counter-clockwise two or three times.
- Your ears, shoulders, wrists, hamstrings, and heels should be in alignment. You can use a wall to help.
- Stand straight, close your eyes, and with your chin touching your upper chest let your body sway forward and backward without moving your feet from the floor. Let your body feel heavy and relaxed. Focus on your breathing.
- Relax the jaw allowing your mouth to drop slightly. Move your jaw around in a circular motion from left to right several times and then from right to left.

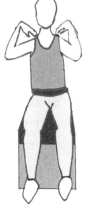

Fig. 12

- Find what works for you, whether it is yoga, meditation, or another technique to help your body relax.

Breathing

Breath involves the coordination of muscles of the ribs together with muscles of the abdomen, a process called muscular antagonism. The muscles of inspiration – the external intercostals and diaphragm – work to create a partial vacuum to help expand the lungs. This breathing is called costo-diaphragmatic breathing and is key for breath support.

Breath support is taught in many different ways. Many teachers use visualization and imagery techniques to help. Below are some techniques that are useful to 'wake up' and strengthen the breathing mechanism. Again, everyone's body is unique and may require personal adjustments best made under the supervision of a good voice teacher. Try the following.

- Stand quietly with good posture.
- Take a quiet breath through the nose to the count of 3, like you are smelling flowers. Keep your arms and shoulders comfortably relaxed. Exhale through your mouth to the count of 4 while keeping your ribs expanded. Over time increase the counts to 6 and then 8. As you become comfortable with the exercise, add a 3-count hold at the top of the inhalation.
- Sense how your body feels while making a /s/ sound. Appreciate how your ribs and sternum feel and how the breath flow is controlled naturally. Now produce the consonant /t/ and feel how the abdominal muscles act.

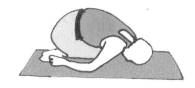

Fig. 13

- • Feel how your abdominal muscles move when breathing in and out in a 'baby position' (Figure 13). Appreciate how your ribs and sternum feel and how the breath flow is controlled naturally. This position will help you to relax and be more in touch with your breathing.

Semi-occluded vocal tract exercises

Semi-occluded vocal tract exercises (SOVTE) can be useful for voice recovery and are good for warm-ups and cool-downs. They must be done gently and without discomfort. Any pain suggests you are doing things incorrectly or something might be wrong.

Semi-occluded vocal tract exercises (SOVTE) are vocal exercises performed by creating a partial blockage of the vocal tract, typically within the oral cavity or at the level of the lips. The blockage causes increased resistance to the flow of air and likely increases interaction between the vocal tract and the vocal folds (feedback between the source and the filter of the sound). In addition to feeling increased resistance to air flow, the vocalist will feel a sensation of tissue vibration throughout the facial structures as the sound production becomes more efficient.

There are a number of different thoughts about how exactly these exercises work or are beneficial, but they are a valuable tool for training, warming up, cooling down the voice, and for voice recovery. Ultimately, they help produce voice more efficiently – in other words, better quality sound with less trauma to the vocal folds.

SOVTE have been used for many years. Traditional ways of performing SOVTE include performing using lip trills, tongue trills, and humming. Simple straws and tubes can also be used which elongate the vocal tract. Sensations will vary depending on the method used. Larger straws, such as those you might find with a smoothie, have less resistance and are likely more appropriate when vocal fatigue is present and voice recovery is the main goal. In addition, larger straws are more appropriate for novices without a lot of voice training. When a large straw is used, an /oo/ vowel is appropriate when making sound. When a smaller straw (such as a stirring straw) is used, a fricative, such as a /b/ sound should be made. The depth of the water can be altered. Less water will also provide lower resistance and thus require less effort.

Much has been written on SOVTE. In the box below are a few references. We encourage you to explore further if you are interested.

Titze. 2006. Voice training and therapy with a semi-occluded vocal tract: rationale and scientific underpinnings. *Journal of Speech, Language and Hearing Research* 49(2): 448–59.

Bele. 2005. Artifically lengthened and constricted vocal tract in vocal training methods. *Logopedics Phoniatrics Vocology* 30: 34–40.

Laukkanen, Lindholm & Vilkman. 1995. Phonation into a tube as a voice training method. Acoustic and physiologic observations. *Folia Phoniatrica et Logopaedica* 47:331–38.

Below are some exercises to try. Remember, if you are recovering the voice, use a large straw and start with bubbles with no sound. Silicone tubes, larger than a normal straw, are also useful (Figure 14). You should feel no strain or discomfort. If you do, you should stop and seek supervision. One nice thing about doing the SOVTE exercises with a straw is that you can do them quietly anywhere, anytime.

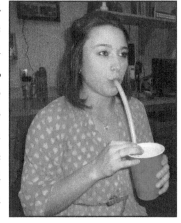

Figure 14

Bubbles with no sound

1. Sit in a relaxed posture upright in a chair or standing. Make sure the face, neck, shoulders, upper back and chest are all relaxed.
2. Place the straw into the cup of water or a water bottle.
   a. The water should be about two fingers deep in the cup.
   b. Hold the cup near the body; make sure not to tense your shoulders while holding the cup.
3. Place the straw in your mouth in front of or between your incisor teeth and your tongue.
   a. Close your lips around the straw.
   b. Keep your tongue relaxed and slightly touching the straw.
4. Take a deep breath in.
   a. Inhale from your nose while your mouth is closed around the straw, like yawning with your mouth closed, and think of the position of the vowel /oo/. Make no sound. Feel the vibration in your cheeks.
   b. On inhalation, feel your diaphragm lower and ribcage expand.
5. Exhale by blowing air through the straw, making bubbles in the water.
   a. Remember to maintain your relaxed posture.
   b. On exhalation, abdominal muscles should retract inwards.
   c. Continue to blow bubbles until you feel the need to inhale again.
6. Repeat (at least 10 times each).
7. Feel the vibrations in your cheeks during this exercise.
8. Speak short phrases with this new sense of facial vibration immediately following the exercise.

Bubbles with sound

Follow steps 1–3 from above.

4.   Create a sustained sound through the straw, making bubbles in the water.

   a.   Remember to maintain your relaxed posture.

   b.   On exhalation, your lower abdomen should retract inwards.

   c.   Continue to make the sound until you feel the need to inhale.

5.   Sustain each pitch (low, medium, and high) using a medium intensity level (at least 10 times each pitch) with the sound /oo/.

6.   Continue to make the sound while blowing the bubbles, sliding your pitch from low to high (glissando). Not too heavy, not too light. Remember to use good breath support.

7.   Sing 'Happy Birthday' or another familiar song through the straw while blowing bubbles on the sustained vowel.

8.   The more advanced singer can try additional tasks such as scales, arpeggios using staccato techniques, and *messa di voce* exercises.

Humming, lip trills, and tongue trills are also SOVTE and can be used for warm-ups and cool-downs as well. Some are described below in the 'resonance' section.

Resonance

When the onset of voice is coordinated with exhalation and the vocal tract is prepared to enhance the harmonic spectrum, the voice will flow and ring beautifully. The full potential of the voice will be reached. Each individual must discover how to use his or her body's resonators to the fullest. One can 'play' with his or her voice to try to find how to 'place' the voice to maximize resonation. SOVTE exercises may help with this. How one uses the resonators differs for each individual and for different genres of music. The resonators can also be used to assist with producing character voices without straining the vocal folds. Working with an appropriate voice teacher is quite helpful.

Below are some techniques that can help discover, 'wake-up', and maximize the potential of the resonators. Some of these exercises are for more advanced singers. Feel free to skip them if they do not make sense to you. On the other hand, using the singing voice even for the non-singer can be helpful for overall vocal health.

Resonance exercises

- Perform several voluntary yawns in an easy relax manner. Easy relaxed yawning promotes relaxation of the vocal mechanism.
- Breathe in, hold your breath for the count of 3 and ease the air out slowly with pursed lips.
- Yawn and do a gentle sigh with expiration.
- Bring the lips gently together as if humming [m]. Place the tip of the tongue easily behind the upper teeth as if singing [n]. Hum using this combination of [m] and [n]. Experiment in mid-range with random humming sounds, single pitches, and gentle glissandos. Appreciate the sensations in the nose and face. Humming is a type of SOVTE and is useful for warming up, cooling down, and improving resonation.
- Hum with [m] and [n], but extend each one to an /oo/ (carry it into a 'moo' or 'noo'). Again, experiment in a comfortable range, single pitches, then glissandos (sliding from low pitch to high pitch).
- Hum one of your favorite songs in a comfortable range.
- Sustain a sound in a single pitch in mid-voice, first hummed pianissimo and then sung with gradual crescendo on a succession

of vowels that grow increasingly brighter: [u–o–a]. If the vowel is truly unified, somewhere in the [a] an overtone (or sometimes two) emerges as a result of the vowel unification. For optimum sound, think in this order: Breathe, Sing, Sustain, Release.

· Perform one-octave glissandos from high to low using /he/ and /mu/.

· Try humming other vocal exercises you may know, e.g. scales and arpeggios. See how tongue and lip trills feel, too!

The nose

Noses big and small are important resonators. Keeping them clean and open is important. If you have significant nasal obstruction, you should consider seeing an otolaryngologist (ENT). Below are some 'nasal exercises' that can be useful.

Nasal exercises

1. Close one nostril and inhale with the other for the count of 4, hold for 4, and exhale for 4. Then do the other.

2. Do alternate nostril breathing.

   a. Use your right thumb to close off your right nostril (index finger between your eyebrows).

   b. Inhale slowly through your left nostril.

   c. Pause for a second.

   d. Now close your left nostril with your middle finger and release your thumb off your nostril.

   e. Exhale through your right nostril.

   f. Now, inhale through your right nostril.

   g. Pause.

   h. Use your thumb to close your right nostril.

   i. Breathe out through your left nostril

    j.   This is one round. Start slowly with one or two rounds and gradually increase. Never force. Sit quietly for a few moments after you have finished.

3.   Hum as you close one nostril and breathe through the other. Repeat this several times. Feel the vibration in your nose and face.

4.   Read a paragraph and try to appreciate the same sensations.

Articulation

Articulation is important to the performer. Voiced consonants engage the vocal folds, and poor technique during speaking or singing can cause vocal trauma and lead to poor vocal quality. The key to healthy articulation is maintaining relaxation of the jaw, tongue, and lips, and using the resonators efficiently.

Tongue relaxation

Your tongue is a big muscle and needs to relax. This helps with articulation. Excessive tension in the tongue can affect the vocal tract and therefore affect resonation and the quality of the sound. Tongue tension can also cause tension of other neck musculature and contribute to trauma of the vocal folds. Below are some simple things you can do to help your tongue relax. Sit or stand upright with good posture while performing these tasks.

Tongue relaxation exercises

- Stick out your tongue as far as possible and hold it for 5 seconds before resting.
- Do just the opposite by retracting your tongue inside your mouth and holding it at the roof of your mouth for 3 seconds before relaxing.

55

- Make a clicking noise by moving your tongue up and down against your hard palate,
- Pull your tongue out and down with your fingers (wash your hands first ☺). You can use a gauze.
- Sustain a note in a comfortable range on /hee/ while holding your tongue out.
- For those who read music, follow exercises A, B, and C while holding your tongue out. You may adjust the starting notes for your range.

A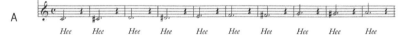

B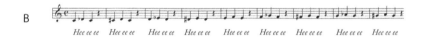

C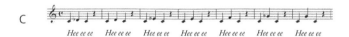

- Let the tongue go back inside your mouth and then do a fake yawn to open the back of the mouth.
- Hum; then try speaking.
- You should feel a full 'open' sensation of the tongue and the sound should feel free and forward.
- Speak short phrases with this new sense of opening immediately following the exercises, or try to sing.
- Do these exercises once or twice throughout the day, before performances or rehearsal when you feel tension/strain at the back of the tongue.
- Tongue twisters will get the tongue muscles warmed up. These should be done with as little tension within the tongue as possible. Some examples are below:

 Many million men are married in the month of May.

 Peter Piper picked a peck of pickled peppers.

A peck of pickled peppers Peter Piper picked.

If Peter Piper picked a peck of pickled peppers

Where's the peck of pickled peppers Peter Piper picked?

Avoiding the hard glottal attack

The hard glottal attack involves excessive force during the initiation of voice. The vocal folds forcefully close, potentially causing injury. This often occurs with words beginning with a vowel. Good breath support, relaxation of the throat, lower jaw, and back of the tongue are all very important for eliminating glottal attacks

One can train soft initiation of voice with monosyllables that start with /h/. One can also place a /h/ in front of words that start with a vowel. One can then try to take the sensation of soft initiation and use it when saying the word without the /h/. Alternating such words with and without the /h/ is a useful exercise. Below are some examples:

heat $\leftrightarrow$ eat   heel $\leftrightarrow$ eel

hire $\leftrightarrow$ ire   hold $\leftrightarrow$ old

Try these sentences which alternate words beginning with /h/ with words beginning with vowels. Concentrate on soft initiation of sound.

1. Helen heals her hand every evening.
2. Every evening Helen heals her hand.

Lastly, linking words can help avoid the hard glottal attack. For example:

1. Helen adores singing. Try linking 'Helen adores' to make 'Helenadores'.
2. Anna always enjoyed parties. Try linking the first three words: 'Annaalwaysenjoyed'.

For more reading on the 'hard glottal attack', we refer you to Edith Skinner's *Speak with Distinction* (1990, Applause Theater Book Publishing).

Whoa, now take a breath and relax. Hopefully you found this chapter useful. Some of these exercises may not suit you. That's fine. Take away what you feel is helpful. However, all of the points made here – warming-up, cooling down, good posture, finding ways to improve your breath support, and resonance – are all useful for improving vocal quality and maintaining vocal health. Again, a book cannot replace good vocal training, but we hope these tips and techniques are useful for you.

Appendix I
A bit of anatomy

This appendix is for those of you who want a bit more detail about the larynx and the structure of the vocal folds. It is not necessary for the overall purpose of this handbook, but I thought I would throw it in for the more adventurous readers.

Muscles of the larynx

The illustration below shows all the small muscles within the larynx. The simultaneous action of all these muscles determines the position and tension on the vocal folds. The cricothyroid muscle is the main muscle that elongates or stretches the vocal fold. Paralysis of this muscle will affect a person's ability to hit higher pitches. This muscle is activated by the superior laryngeal nerve. All the other muscles are activated by the recurrent laryngeal nerve.

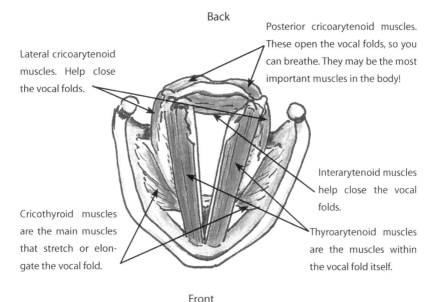

Back

Posterior cricoarytenoid muscles. These open the vocal folds, so you can breathe. They may be the most important muscles in the body!

Lateral cricoarytenoid muscles. Help close the vocal folds.

Interarytenoid muscles help close the vocal folds.

Cricothyroid muscles are the main muscles that stretch or elongate the vocal fold.

Thyroarytenoid muscles are the muscles within the vocal fold itself.

Front

Layers of the vocal fold

This illustration represents a slice through the vocal fold. It shows the different layers of the fold: the deepest layer is the thyroarytenoid muscle. The next layer is the vocal ligament. If this layer is injured during surgery, tremendous scarring typically occurs resulting in poor voice quality. The next layer is Reinke's space (also called the superficial lamina propria). This is the voice's best friend, as it is the most pliable layer of the vocal fold. If it is lost, the outer layer, or epithelium, will get tacked down to the vocal ligament and become stiffer. To date, we have no dependable way of replacing lost Reinke's space, so care must be taken to preserve it by practising good vocal hygiene.

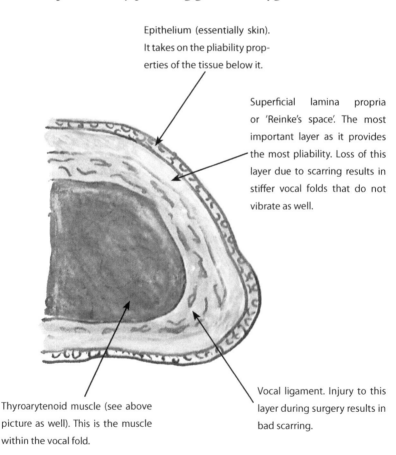

Epithelium (essentially skin). It takes on the pliability properties of the tissue below it.

Superficial lamina propria or 'Reinke's space'. The most important layer as it provides the most pliability. Loss of this layer due to scarring results in stiffer vocal folds that do not vibrate as well.

Thyroarytenoid muscle (see above picture as well). This is the muscle within the vocal fold.

Vocal ligament. Injury to this layer during surgery results in bad scarring.

In this image of the larynx the blue double-arrow lies along the thyroarytenoid muscle. The black double arrow lies over the vocal ligament. Reinke's space is not discernible, because it is a clear thin layer that covers the entire vocal fold. You cannot see the other muscles of the larynx because they are covered by tissue.

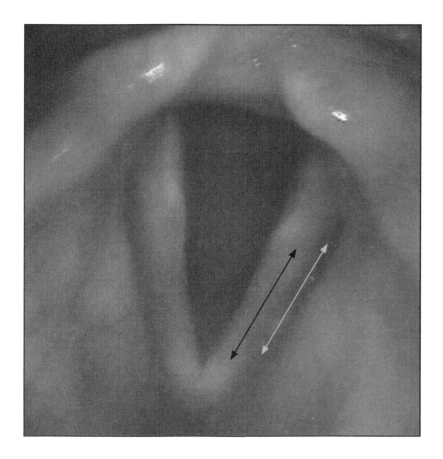

Appendix II
Twenty-five tips for a healthy voice

1. Avoid shouting.

2. Avoid talking in loud environments (e.g. bars, parties, restaurants, airplanes). Wear earplugs as that will help you hear yourself better. Think twice about jumping on your cell phone when you get in the car.

3. Drink plenty of water. Pee pale.

4. Avoid clearing your throat (swallow or sip water instead) and suppress cough when possible.

5. Avoid bearing down and grunting during weight-lifting, exercise, and other activities (even sex).

6. Do not smoke and avoid second-hand smoke. Avoid other irritating inhalants as well. Wear a mask in the work environment if there are fumes.

7. Avoid foods and behaviors that are irritating or stimulate acid reflux.

8. Avoid excessive alcohol. It is bad for reflux *and* your judgement. It might lead to loud talking and singing heavy metal tunes which you cannot quite handle . . .

9. Avoid forceful whispering.

10. Take frequent voice naps. Do not use your voice when it is not necessary.

11. Check with your doctor about which of your medications may affect your voice and beware homeopathic medications.

12. Get plenty of rest. Recover from jet lag before a performance.

13. Get voice training. You can train your speaking *and* your singing voice. Continue training throughout your career if possible.

14. Beware of surgeries that might injure the nerves to your vocal folds (e.g. neck and chest surgeries). Also, if you require surgery with a general anesthetic, tell the anesthesiologist to use the smallest endotracheal tube possible. Also tell him or her how important your voice is to you, and to *please* be careful around your vocal folds.

15. Beware of character voices and 'stage screams'. Make sure you do them in a healthy way.

16. Speak in a comfortable pitch range.

17. Warm-up and cool-down. Remember good posture and breath support.

18. Sing age- and voice-appropriate repertoire.

19. Use monitors and amplification when possible.

20. Understand the effects of medication on your voice. When possible, avoid medications which thin the blood (and make you more susceptible to vocal fold hemorrhage), dry you out, or irritate the vocal folds.

21. Go home and be quiet after a performance. Resist excessive talking to adoring fans, family, groupies, etc.

22. *Do not ignore changes in vocal quality.* If you get hoarse and can rest your voice for a few days, do so. If it returns to normal, great. If not, seek evaluation. Any hoarseness over two weeks always warrants evaluation. The performer should have an even lower threshold for seeking out a voice team.

23. Know where to seek help and what makes for an adequate evaluation of the voice and vocal folds.

24. Read this book again.

25. Career longevity is dependent on maintaining a healthy voice. Make wise decisions and protect yourself.

Also, see 'Rules for a cold' in Chapter 4!

Appendix III
Your one stop vocal health roadmap

This is a simple algorithm for some guidance if you develop hoarseness. This is not an exact science. Some judgement on your part is required. If you have any symptoms besides voice change which are concerning, such as neurologic symptoms, throat pain, high fever , trouble swallowing, or trouble breathing, see a doctor immediately.

Note 1: A sudden change in voice quality during voice use is highly suggestive of a vocal fold hemorrhage. A voice evaluation is highly recommended prior to continued voice use.

Note 2: A voice evaluation would ideally be performed by a 'voice team' equipped with videostroboscopy. (See chapter 5.)

Note 3: Medical management could include medications and voice therapy.

Note 4: 'Normal' means 'normal', not 'acceptable'. If there is still some difference in your vocal quality after 2 weeks, seek a voice evaluation.

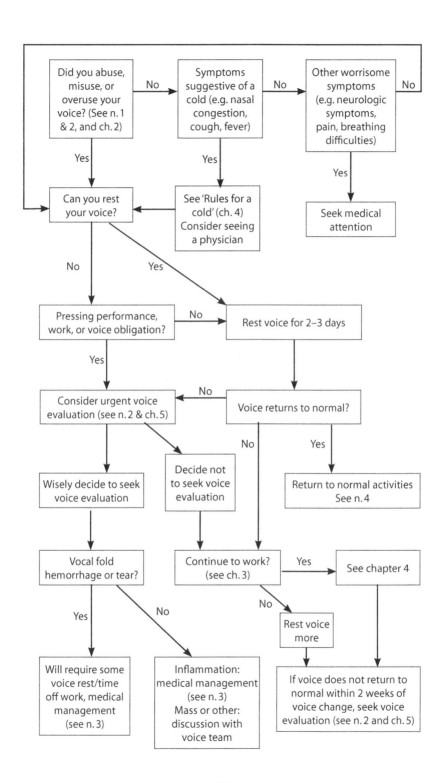

Afterword

The keys to maintaining a healthy voice are:

1. Prevention of vocal injury.
2. Recognition of vocal injury.
3. Appropriate and timely management of vocal injury to avoid long-term sequelae, particularly vocal fold SCAR.

The goal of this handbook is to provide a guide to remind you how to do all do all three. Whether you are a singer at the Metropolitan Opera, a Broadway performer, singer in your church choir, high school teacher, sales manager, doctor, lawyer, or PTA president, your voice is the motor that drives your career, passion, or both. It is an expression of your soul, as well as your source of livelihood. It is up to you to make sure that it remains healthy and functioning properly. There is no one better to recognize a change in your voice quality than you, yourself. Now you have the tools to know what that change in quality might mean, and what you should do about it.

Although many voice problems will resolve on their own, some will not. Further misuse or abuse may lead to more complications and difficulty in regaining your normal voice. Any voice change lasting longer than two weeks demands attention. For those of you with occupations or hobbies requiring pristine vocal quality, an even lower threshold for seeking attention should be maintained. We cannot emphasize enough how many people we see at our voice center on a daily basis who regret not seeking attention sooner. Many say the same thing, that they assumed they had 'laryngitis' and it would get better on its own. When voice problems are identified early, they can often be treated with conservative (non-surgical) management. Even if surgery is required, earlier recognition and treatment will provide the best chance for voice recovery.

It is up to you to know when and from whom to seek attention. It is up to you to recognize who is best prepared to evaluate and treat you. Are they a voice specialist, e.g. a laryngologist or voice pathologist? Do they work as a 'voice team' at a 'voice center'? Do they have the tools to adequately evaluate you? *The Vocal Pitstop* will prompt you on when and where to turn to put you on the road to voice recovery, maintenance, and longevity. Keep it by your side – make it easy to stop in regularly for a Vocal Pitstop.

Author biographies

Adam D. Rubin, M.D.

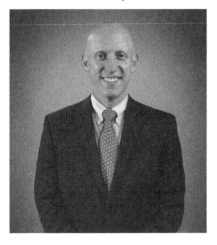

Adam Rubin has had a life-long passion for the human voice. Before attending medical school, he was a professional actor and singer, performing in musicals and plays at off-Broadway and regional theaters, as well as in a national tour. He was a member of the Actors Equity Association, Screen Actors Guild, and American Federation of Television and Radio Artists. He is also a violinist and has dabbled in song writing.

Currently a laryngologist and Director of the Lakeshore Professional Voice Center in St. Clair Shores, Michigan, he graduated *summa cum laude* from Yale College with degrees in Theater Studies and Economics. He received his medical doctorate from Harvard Medical School. Following his residency in Otolaryngology-Head and Neck Surgery at the University of Michigan, he completed a fellowship in Laryngology and Care of the Professional Voice under the direction of Robert T. Sataloff, M.D., D.M.A., at the American Institute for Voice and Ear Research.

In addition to his clinical and artistic expertise, Dr. Rubin is active in voice research. He has written many book chapters and numerous scientific articles published in major otolaryngology journals. He is a frequent presenter at national and international meetings. He is a member of the American Academy of Otolaryngology, American Laryngological Association, Triological Society, and the Michigan Otolaryngology Society. He has academic appointments at the University of Michigan, Michigan State University, and the Oakland University William Beaumont School of Medicine. One of his biggest joys is hosting an annual World Voice Day concert every April, in which he and many of his patients sing and celebrate voice recovery. Most importantly, he is a loving husband and father of two wonderful children.

Maria Cristina A. Jackson-Menaldi, Ph.D.

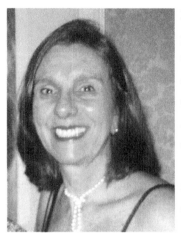

Dr. Jackson-Menaldi has worked as a voice pathologist and singing voice specialist for over 40 years. She and Dr. Daniel Megler created the Lakeshore Professional Voice Center in 1991, which she has co-directed with Dr. Adam Rubin for the last ten years. She is an adjunct professor at Wayne State University School of Medicine in Detroit, MI. She holds master degrees in speech language pathology, audiology, and choir directing from the University of Museo Social Argentino, Buenos Aires, Argentina; solfeggio and piano from the National Music Conservatory of Buenos Aires; and a post-doctoral degree in general phonetics from the University of Sorbonne Nouvelle, Paris France. She has worked as a professor at the University of Salvador, Museo Social Argentino, University of Buenos Aires, the National Music Conservatory, and Teatro Colon in Buenos Aires, as well as the Music Conservatory and the University of the Sorbonne, in Paris, France. She also has worked internationally as a choir director and in-house voice pathologist for opera houses and music conservatories. She continues to lecture internationally.

Dr. Jackson-Menaldi has written numerous scientific articles and book chapters. She has written the books *La Voz Patologia* and *La Voz Normal*, published by Editorial Medica, Panamericana. She is a well-known leader in the professional voice community.

Daniel Cascardo

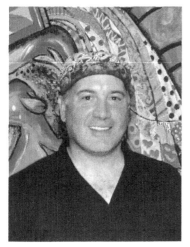

Challenging the viewer to be inspired and use his imagination is the goal of Daniel Cascardo, a nationally recognized visual artist and Michigan native.His approach to art is to interpret life in a very positive and thought provoking manner through the use of uninhibited brush strokes, bright colors, patterns, symbols, and various forms of nature – including fantastic birds and fish – that let your imagination soar.

Currently a resident of Royal Oak, Mich., Cascardo maintains a private studio and travels to a variety of locations to work with schools, corporations, and other organizations to engage individuals in team building experiences through the use of art. Among the honors Cascardo has received, he won the Starbucks Artist Recognition Award in 2006 for a mural that was created for the speciality coffee retailer's Michigan Avenue store in west Dearborn, Mich. Cascardo was awarded the Mayors Arts Award for his art in 2011. He was part of a national promotional campaign for True Religion Fragrances sold in Macy department stores across the country. He recently received the peoples choice award for a POP up gallery in Dearborn, Michigan.

Cascardo works in a variety of media including canvas, wood, glass, and textiles. He showcases his personal style and examples of work in different art media on his website, www.danielcascardo.com. Upbeat rhythmic music, color photos, video clips, a gallery, shop, and blog are all used to create an interactive experience for online visitors as well as to help them be entertained and to gain a feeling and appreciation for Cascardo's free flowing, abstract style.

His website includes an online shop to purchase prints, t-shirts, and other items that appeal to people who like his work and have a more limited budget. Cascardo enjoys hearing from visitors who visit his website and learn how his art can be applied to their lives.

Melissa Errico

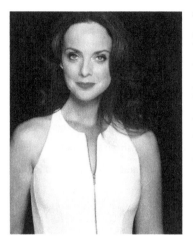

Tony-Award Nominee Melissa Errico is a Broadway force whose talents span the stage, music, and the screen.

Praised by critics and audiences alike, the *New York Times* proclaimed Errico 'The Voice of Enchantment' with her performances described as 'commanding', 'incandescent', and 'beguiling and enigmatic'. She most recently completed her run as Clara in the highly-acclaimed 2013 Classic Theater Company revival of *Passion* by Stephen Sondheim, earning her sixth Drama Desk Award nomination. She also appeared in the lauded *Kurt Weil on Broadway*, reprising her work as Venus in celebration of the release of the first-ever recording of 'One Touch of Venus'.

Influenced by the great Dames of the stage, Errico interrupted her studies at Yale to accept the iconic role of Cosette in the first national touring company of *Les Misérables*. After returning and completing her degree, she debuted on Broadway in *Anna Karenina*, later singing the epomonyous role on the 2007 cast album. Her Broadway credits include the revival of *My Fair Lady*, in which she played Eliza Doolittle, *High Society*, *Amour* (Tony nomination for Best Leading Actress in a Musical), *Dracula, the Musical* and *White Christmas*. In 2004, she starred in the wildly successful off-Broadway production of *Finian's Rainbow*, winning an array of awards, and made an acclaimed recording of that show. Melissa has also earned Drama Desk Award nominations for each of her starring roles in non-musical roles in such great plays as *The Importance of Being Earnest*, *Major Barbara*, and *Candida*. She has also starred in Wally Shawn's *Aunt Dan and Lemon* with Lili Taylor and in the US premier of *Gift of the Gorgon* opposite Alec Baldwin. She was selected by Stephen Sondheim to star in *Sunday in The Park With George* at The Kennedy Center.

Errico's command of both the small and silver screen is evident with roles on *The Good Wife*, *Law and Order*, *Blue Bloods*, *Central Park West*, and others. She has also appeared opposite film stars Angelina Jolie in *Life or Something Like It*, Dennis Quaid in *Frequency*, and Kyra Sedgewick in *Loverboy*, directed by Kevin Bacon.

Proving her vocal talents transcend the stage, Errico has released several albums to date; most recently collaborating with noted film/jazz/pop composer Michel Legrand and legendary producer Phil Ramone on *Legrand Affair*. Her experience surrounding the project inspired her published essay entitled 'Musing'. Her debut solo album *Blue Like That* produced by industry legend Arif Mardin, and follow up album *Lullabies and Wildflowers*, also garnered critical acclaim.

Errico has an extensive concert history including appearances at The Rose Auditorium Lincoln Center, Dizzy's Jazz Club, The Cafe Carlyle, Joe's Pub, The Kennedy Center, and Avery Fisher Hall, and throughout the country with esteemed symphonies such as the National Symphony Orchestra and The Cleveland Orchestra. In 2008, she made a successful London concert debut at the Palladium with Angela Lansbury and the Royal Philharmonic Orchestra.

Melissa Errico lives in Manhattan with her husband Patrick McEnroe and their three daughters.

She is currently shooting the new Cinemax series *The Knick* starring Clive Owen, directed and produced by Stephen Soderbergh, which airs in 2014.

Ron Livingston

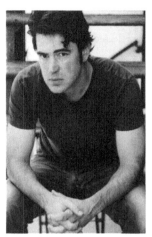

Ron Livingston is a professional actor and once-in-a-while singer, best known for projects like *Swingers*, *Office Space*, *Band of Brothers*, *Sex and the City*, and *Boardwalk Empire*. He most recently appeared as Elvis Presley in a performance that required dusting off a high B-natural. Ron lives in Los Angeles, California with his wife Rosemarie and daughter Gracie.

Lightning Source UK Ltd.
Milton Keynes UK
UKOW06f0000070514

231221UK00001B/2/P